PLANT BASED COOKBOOK 2022

MOUTH-WATERING RECIPES

FOR A HEALTHY LIFE

MIKE BOLT

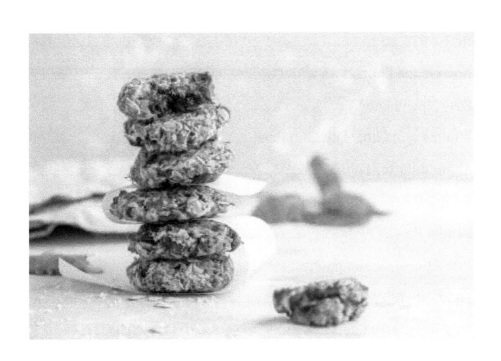

Table of Contents

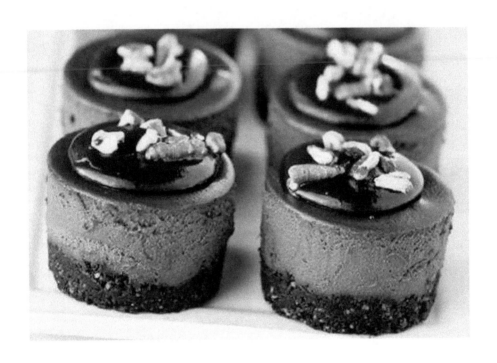

Introduction

It is only until recently that more and more people are starting to embrace the plant-based diet lifestyle. As to what exactly has drawn tens of millions of people into this lifestyle is debatable. However, there is growing evidence demonstrating that following a primarily plant-based diet lifestyle leads to better weight control and general health, free of many chronic diseases. What are the Health Benefits of a Plant-Based Diet? As it turns out, eating plant-based is one of the healthiest diets in the world. Healthy vegan diets include plenty of fresh products, whole grains, legumes, and healthy fats such as seeds and nuts. They are abundant with antioxidants, minerals, vitamins, and dietary fiber. Current scientific researches pointed out that higher consumption of plant-based foods is associated with a lower risk of mortality from conditions such as cardiovascular disease, type 2 diabetes, hypertension, and obesity. Vegan eating plans often rely heavily on healthy staples, avoiding animal products that are loaded with antibiotics, additives, and hormones. Plus, consuming a higher proportion of essential amino acids with animal protein can be damaging to human health. Since animal products contain much 8 more fat than plant-based foods, it's not a shocker that studies have shown that meat-eaters have nine times the obesity rate of vegans. This leads us to the next point, one of the greatest benefits of the vegan diet – weight loss. While many people choose to live a vegan life for ethical reasons, the diet itself can help you achieve your weight loss goals. If you're struggling to shift pounds, you may want to consider trying a plant-based diet. How exactly? As a vegan, you will reduce the number of high-calorie foods such as full-fat dairy products, fatty fish, pork and other cholesterol containing foods such as eggs. Try replacing such foods with high fiber and protein-rich alternatives that will keep you fuller longer. The key is focusing on nutrient-dense, clean and natural foods and avoid empty calories such as sugar, saturated fats, and highly processed foods. Here are a few tricks that help me maintain my weight on the vegan diet for years. I eat vegetables as a main course; I consume good fats in moderation – a good fat such as olive oil does not make you fat; I exercise regularly and cook at home. Enjoy!

DESSERTS

Homemade Chocolates with Coconut and Raisins

(Ready in about 10 minutes + chilling time | Servings 20)

Per serving : Calories: 130; Fat: 9.1g; Carbs: 12.1g; Protein: 1.3g

Ingredients

1/2 cup cacao butter, melted

1/3 cup peanut butter

1/4 cup agave syrup

A pinch of grated nutmeg

A pinch of coarse salt

1/2 teaspoon vanilla extract

1 cup dried coconut, shredded

6 ounces dark chocolate, chopped

3 ounces raisins

Directions

Thoroughly combine all the ingredients, except for the chocolate, in a mixing bowl.

Spoon the mixture into molds. Leave to set hard in a cool place.

Melt the dark chocolate in your microwave. Pour in the melted chocolate until the fillings are covered. Leave to set hard in a cool place.

Enjoy!

Easy Mocha Fudge

(Ready in about 1 hour 10 minutes | Servings 20)

Per serving : Calories: 105; Fat: 5.6g; Carbs: 12.9g; Protein: 1.1g

Ingredients

1 cup cookies, crushed

1/2 cup almond butter

1/4 cup agave nectar

6 ounces dark chocolate, broken into chunks

1 teaspoon instant coffee

A pinch of grated nutmeg

A pinch of salt

Directions

Line a large baking sheet with parchment paper.

Melt the chocolate in your microwave and add in the remaining ingredients; stir to combine well.

Scrape the batter into a parchment-lined baking sheet. Place it in your freezer for at least 1 hour to set.

Cut into squares and serve. Bon appétit!

Almond and Chocolate Chip Bars

(Ready in about 40 minutes | Servings 10)

Per serving : Calories: 295; Fat: 17g; Carbs: 35.2g; Protein: 1.7g

Ingredients

1/2 cup almond butter

1/4 cup coconut oil, melted

1/4 cup agave syrup

1 teaspoon vanilla extract

1/4 teaspoon sea salt

1/4 teaspoon grated nutmeg

1/2 teaspoon ground cinnamon

2 cups almond flour

1/4 cup flaxseed meal

1 cup vegan chocolate, cut into chunks

1 1/3 cups almonds, ground

2 tablespoons cacao powder

1/4 cup agave syrup

Directions

In a mixing bowl, thoroughly combine the almond butter, coconut oil, 1/4 cup of agave syrup, vanilla, salt, nutmeg and cinnamon.

Gradually stir in the almond flour and flaxseed meal and stir to combine. Add in the chocolate chunks and stir again.

In a small mixing bowl, combine the almonds, cacao powder and agave syrup. Now, spread the ganache onto the cake. Freeze for about 30 minutes, cut into bars and serve well chilled. Enjoy!

Almond Butter Cookies

(Ready in about 45 minutes | Servings 10)

Per serving : Calories: 197; Fat: 15.8g; Carbs: 12.5g; Protein: 2.1g

Ingredients

3/4 cup all-purpose flour

1/2 teaspoon baking soda

1/4 teaspoon kosher salt

1 flax egg

1/4 cup coconut oil, at room temperature

2 tablespoons almond milk

1/2 cup brown sugar

1/2 cup almond butter

1/2 teaspoon ground cinnamon

1/2 teaspoon vanilla

Directions

In a mixing bowl, combine the flour, baking soda and salt.

In another bowl, combine the flax egg, coconut oil, almond milk, sugar, almond butter, cinnamon and vanilla. Stir the wet mixture into the dry ingredients and stir until well combined.

Place the batter in your refrigerator for about 30 minutes. Shape the batter into small cookies and arrange them on a parchment-lined cookie pan.

Bake in the preheated oven at 350 degrees F for approximately 12 minutes. Transfer the pan to a wire rack to cool at room temperature. Bon appétit!

Peanut Butter Oatmeal Bars

(Ready in about 25 minutes | Servings 20)

Per serving : Calories: 161; Fat: 10.3g; Carbs: 17.5g; Protein: 2.9g

Ingredients

1 cup vegan butter

3/4 cup coconut sugar

2 tablespoons applesauce

1 ¾ cups old-fashioned oats

1 teaspoon baking soda

A pinch of sea salt

A pinch of grated nutmeg

1 teaspoon pure vanilla extract

1 cup oat flour

1 cup all-purpose flour

Directions

Begin by preheating your oven to 350 degrees F.

In a mixing bowl, thoroughly combine the dry ingredients. In another bowl, combine the wet ingredients.

Then, stir the wet mixture into the dry ingredients; mix to combine well.

Spread the batter mixture in a parchment-lined square baking pan. Bake in the preheated oven for about 20 minutes. Enjoy!

Vanilla Halvah Fudge

(Ready in about 10 minutes + chilling time | Servings 16)

Per serving : Calories: 106; Fat: 9.8g; Carbs: 4.5g; Protein: 1.4g

Ingredients

1/2 cup cocoa butter

1/2 cup tahini

8 dates, pitted

1/4 teaspoon ground cloves

A pinch of grated nutmeg

A pinch coarse salt

1 teaspoon vanilla extract

Directions

Line a square baking pan with parchment paper.

Mix the ingredients until everything is well incorporated.

Scrape the batter into the parchment-lined pan. Place in your freezer until ready to serve. Bon appétit!

Raw Chocolate Mango Pie

(Ready in about 10 minutes + chilling time | Servings 16)

Per serving : Calories: 196; Fat: 16.8g; Carbs: 14.1g; Protein: 1.8g

Ingredients

Avocado layer:

3 ripe avocados, pitted and peeled

A pinch of sea salt

A pinch of ground anise

1/2 teaspoon vanilla paste

2 tablespoons coconut milk

5 tablespoons agave syrup

1/3 cup cocoa powder

Crema layer:

1/3 cup almond butter

1/2 cup coconut cream

1 medium mango, peeled

1/2 coconut flakes

2 tablespoons agave syrup

Directions

In your food processor, blend the avocado layer until smooth and uniform; reserve.

Then, blend the other layer in a separate bowl. Spoon the layers in a lightly oiled baking pan.

Transfer the cake to your freezer for about 3 hours. Store in your freezer. Bon appétit!

Chocolate N'ice Cream

(Ready in about 10 minutes | Servings 1)

Per serving : Calories: 349; Fat: 2.8; Carbs: 84.1g; Protein: 4.8g

Ingredients

2 frozen bananas, peeled and sliced

2 tablespoons coconut milk

1 teaspoon carob powder

1 teaspoon cocoa powder

A pinch of grated nutmeg

1/8 teaspoon ground cardamom

1/8 teaspoon ground cinnamon

1 tablespoon chocolate curls

Directions

Place all the ingredients in the bowl of your food processor or high-speed blender.

Blitz the ingredients until creamy or until your desired consistency is achieved.

Serve immediately or store in your freezer.

Bon appétit!

Raw Raspberry Cheesecake

(Ready in about 15 minutes + chilling time | Servings 9)

Per serving : Calories: 385; Fat: 22.9; Carbs: 41.1g; Protein: 10.8g

Ingredients

Crust:

2 cups almonds

1 cup fresh dates, pitted

1/4 teaspoon ground cinnamon

Filling:

2 cups raw cashews, soaked overnight and drained

14 ounces blackberries, frozen

1 tablespoon fresh lime juice

1/4 teaspoon crystallized ginger

1 can coconut cream

8 fresh dates, pitted

Directions

In your food processor, blend the crust ingredients until the mixture comes together; press the crust into a lightly oiled springform pan.

Then, blend the filling layer until completely smooth. Spoon the filling onto the crust, creating a flat surface with a spatula.

Transfer the cake to your freezer for about 3 hours. Store in your freezer.

Garnish with organic citrus peel. Bon appétit!

Mini Lemon Tarts

(Ready in about 15 minutes + chilling time | Servings 9)

Per serving : Calories: 257; Fat: 16.5; Carbs: 25.4g; Protein: 4g

Ingredients

1 cup cashews

1 cup dates, pitted

1/2 cup coconut flakes

1/2 teaspoon anise, ground

3 lemons, freshly squeezed

1 cup coconut cream

2 tablespoons agave syrup

Directions

Brush a muffin tin with a nonstick cooking oil.

Blend the cashews, dates, coconut and anise in your food processor or a high-speed blender. Press the crust into the peppered muffin tin.

Then, blend the lemon, coconut cream and agave syrup. Spoon the cream into the muffin tin.

Store in your freezer. Bon appétit!

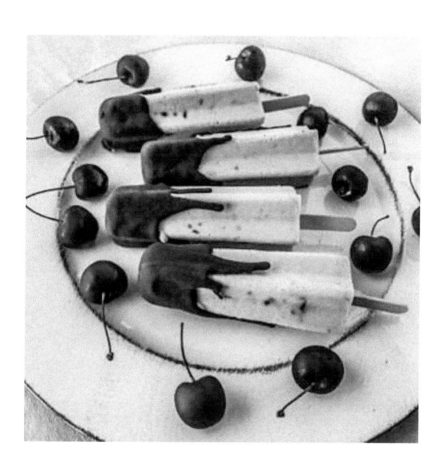

Fluffy Coconut Blondies with Raisins

(Ready in about 30 minutes | Servings 9)

Per serving : Calories: 365; Fat: 18.5; Carbs: 49g; Protein: 2.1g

---

Ingredients

1 cup coconut flour

1 cup all-purpose flour

1/2 teaspoon baking powder

1/4 teaspoon salt

1 cup desiccated coconut, unsweetened

3/4 cup vegan butter, softened

1 ½ cups brown sugar

3 tablespoons applesauce

1/2 teaspoon vanilla extract

1/2 teaspoon ground anise

1 cup raisins, soaked for 15 minutes

Directions

Start by preheating your oven to 350 degrees F. Brush a baking pan with a nonstick cooking oil.

Thoroughly combine the flour, baking powder, salt and coconut. In another bowl, mix the butter, sugar, applesauce, vanilla and anise. Stir the butter mixture into the dry ingredients; stir to combine well.

Fold in the raisins. Press the batter into the prepared baking pan.

Bake for approximately 25 minutes or until it is set in the middle. Place the cake on a wire rack to cool slightly.

Bon appétit!

Easy Chocolate Squares

(Ready in about 1 hour 10 minutes | Servings 20)

Per serving : Calories: 187; Fat: 13.8g; Carbs: 15.1g; Protein: 2.9g

Ingredients

1 cup cashew butter

1 cup almond butter

1/4 cup coconut oil, melted

1/4 cup raw cacao powder

2 ounces dark chocolate

4 tablespoons agave syrup

1 teaspoon vanilla paste

1/4 teaspoon ground cinnamon

1/4 teaspoon ground cloves

Directions

Process all the ingredients in your blender until uniform and smooth.

Scrape the batter into a parchment-lined baking sheet. Place it in your freezer for at least 1 hour to set.

Cut into squares and serve. Bon appétit!

Chocolate and Raisin Cookie Bars

(Ready in about 40 minutes | Servings 10)

Per serving : Calories: 267; Fat: 2.9g; Carbs: 61.1g; Protein: 2.2g

Ingredients

1/2 cup peanut butter, at room temperature

1 cup agave syrup

1 teaspoon pure vanilla extract

1/4 teaspoon kosher salt

2 cups almond flour

1 teaspoon baking soda

1 cup raisins

1 cup vegan chocolate, broken into chunks

Directions

In a mixing bowl, thoroughly combine the peanut butter, agave syrup, vanilla and salt.

Gradually stir in the almond flour and baking soda and stir to combine. Add in the raisins and chocolate chunks and stir again.

Freeze for about 30 minutes and serve well chilled. Enjoy!

Almond Granola Bars

(Ready in about 25 minutes | Servings 12)

Per serving : Calories: 147; Fat: 5.9g; Carbs: 21.7g; Protein: 5.2g

Ingredients

1/2 cup spelt flour

1/2 cup oat flour

1 cup rolled oats

1 teaspoon baking powder

1/2 teaspoon cinnamon

1/2 teaspoon ground cardamom

1/4 teaspoon freshly grated nutmeg

1/8 teaspoon kosher salt

1 cup almond milk

3 tablespoons agave syrup

1/2 cup peanut butter

1/2 cup applesauce

1/2 teaspoon pure almond extract

1/2 teaspoon pure vanilla extract

1/2 cup almonds, slivered

Directions

Begin by preheating your oven to 350 degrees F.

In a mixing bowl, thoroughly combine the flour, oats, baking powder and spices. In another bowl, combine the wet ingredients.

Then, stir the wet mixture into the dry ingredients; mix to combine well. Fold in the slivered almonds.

Scrape the batter mixture into a parchment-lined baking pan. Bake in the preheated oven for about 20 minutes. Let it cool on a wire rack. Cut into bars and enjoy!

Fluffy Coconut Cookies

(Ready in about 40 minutes | Servings 10)

Per serving : Calories: 136; Fat: 7.3g; Carbs: 15.6g; Protein: 1.6g

Ingredients

1/2 cup oat flour

1/2 cup all-purpose flour

1/2 teaspoon baking soda

A pinch of salt

1/4 teaspoon grated nutmeg

1/2 teaspoon ground cloves

1/2 teaspoon ground cinnamon

4 tablespoons coconut oil

2 tablespoons oat milk

1/2 cup coconut sugar

1/2 cup coconut flakes, unsweetened

Directions

In a mixing bowl, combine the flour, baking soda and spices.

In another bowl, combine the coconut oil, oat milk, sugar and coconut. Stir the wet mixture into the dry ingredients and stir until well combined.

Place the batter in your refrigerator for about 30 minutes. Shape the batter into small cookies and arrange them on a parchment-lined cookie pan.

Bake in the preheated oven at 330 degrees F for approximately 10 minutes. Transfer the pan to a wire rack to cool at room temperature. Bon appétit!

Raw Walnut and Berry Cake

(Ready in about 10 minutes + chilling time | Servings 8)

Per serving : Calories: 244; Fat: 10.2g; Carbs: 39g; Protein: 3.8g

Ingredients

Crust:

1 ½ cups walnuts, ground

2 tablespoons maple syrup

1/4 cup raw cacao powder

1/4 teaspoon ground cinnamon

A pinch of coarse salt

A pinch of freshly grated nutmeg

Berry layer:

6 cups mixed berries

2 frozen bananas

1/2 cup agave syrup

Directions

In your food processor, blend the crust ingredients until the mixture comes together; press the crust into a lightly oiled baking pan.

Then, blend the berry layer. Spoon the berry layer onto the crust, creating a flat surface with a spatula.

Transfer the cake to your freezer for about 3 hours. Store in your freezer. Bon appétit!

Chocolate Dream Balls

(Ready in about 10 minutes + chilling time | Servings 8)

Per serving : Calories: 107; Fat: 7.2g; Carbs: 10.8g; Protein: 1.8g

Ingredients

3 tablespoons cocoa powder

8 fresh dates, pitted and soaked for 15 minutes

2 tablespoons tahini, at room temperature

1/2 teaspoon ground cinnamon

1/2 cup vegan chocolate, broken into chunks

1 tablespoon coconut oil, at room temperature

Directions

Add the cocoa powder, dates, tahini and cinnamon to the bowl of your food processor. Process until the mixture forms a ball.

Use a cookie scoop to portion the mixture into 1-ounce portions. Roll the balls and refrigerate them for at least 30 minutes.

Meanwhile, microwave the chocolate until melted; add in the coconut oil and whisk to combine well.

Dip the chocolate balls in the coating and store them in your refrigerator until ready to serve. Bon appétit!

Last-Minute Macaroons

(Ready in about 15 minutes | Servings 10)

Per serving : Calories: 125; Fat: 7.2g; Carbs: 14.3g; Protein: 1.1g

Ingredients

3 cups coconut flakes, sweetened

9 ounces canned coconut milk, sweetened

1 teaspoon ground anise

1 teaspoon vanilla extract

Directions

Begin by preheating your oven to 325 degrees F. Line the cookie sheets with parchment paper.

Thoroughly combine all the ingredients until everything is well incorporated.

Use a cookie scoop to drop mounds of the batter onto the prepared cookie sheets.

Bake for about 11 minutes until they are lightly browned. Bon appétit!

Old-Fashioned Ratafias

(Ready in about 20 minutes | Servings 8)

Per serving : Calories: 272; Fat: 16.2g; Carbs: 28.6g; Protein: 5.8g

Ingredients

2 ounces all-purpose flour

2 ounces almond flour

1 teaspoon baking powder

2 tablespoons applesauce

5 ounces caster sugar

1 ½ ounces vegan butter

4 drops of ratafia essence

Directions

Start by preheating your oven to 330 degrees F. Line a cookie sheet with parchment paper.

Thoroughly combine all the ingredients until everything is well incorporated.

Use a cookie scoop to drop mounds of the batter onto the prepared cookie sheet.

Bake for about 15 minutes until they are lightly browned. Bon appétit!

Jasmine Rice Pudding with Dried Apricots

(Ready in about 20 minutes | Servings 4)

Per serving : Calories: 300; Fat: 2.2g; Carbs: 63.6g; Protein: 5.6g

Ingredients

1 cup jasmine rice, rinsed

1 cup water

1 cup almond milk

1/2 cup brown sugar

A pinch of salt

A pinch of grated nutmeg

1/2 cup dried apricots, chopped

1/4 teaspoon cinnamon powder

1 teaspoon vanilla extract

Directions

Add the rice and water to a saucepan. Cover the saucepan and bring the water to a boil.

Turn the heat to low; let it simmer for another 10 minutes until all the water is absorbed.

Then, add in the remaining ingredients and stir to combine. Let it simmer for 10 minutes more or until the pudding has thickened. Bon appétit!

Everyday Energy Bars

(Ready in about 35 minutes | Servings 16)

Per serving : Calories: 285; Fat: 17.1g; Carbs: 30g; Protein: 5.1g

Ingredients

1 cup vegan butter

1 cup brown sugar

2 tablespoons agave syrup

2 cups old-fashioned oats

1/2 cup almonds, slivered

1/2 cup walnuts, chopped

1/2 cup dried currants

1/2 cup pepitas

Directions

Begin by preheating your oven to 320 degrees F. Line a baking pan with parchment paper or Silpat mat.

Thoroughly combine all the ingredients until everything is well incorporated.

Spread the mixture onto the prepared baking pan using a wide spatula.

Bake for about 33 minutes or until golden brown. Cut into bars using a sharp knife and enjoy!

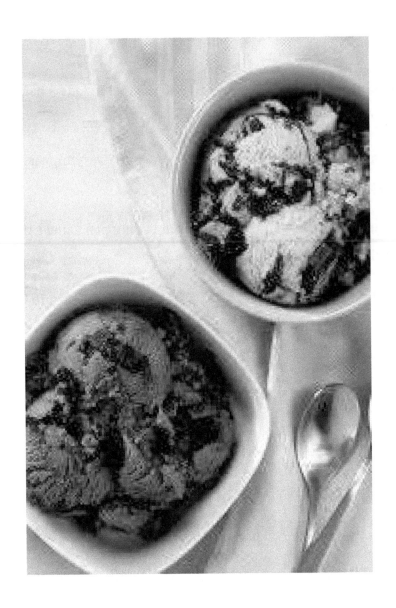

Raw Coconut Ice Cream

(Ready in about 10 minutes + chilling time | Servings 2)

Per serving : Calories: 388; Fat: 7.7g; Carbs: 82g; Protein: 4.8g

Ingredients

4 over-ripe bananas, frozen

4 tablespoons coconut milk

6 fresh dates, pitted

1/4 teaspoon pure coconut extract

1/2 teaspoon pure vanilla extract

1/2 cup coconut flakes

Directions

Place all the ingredients in the bowl of your food processor or high-speed blender.

Blitz the ingredients until creamy or until your desired consistency is achieved.

Serve immediately or store in your freezer.

Bon appétit!

Chocolate Hazelnut Fudge

(Ready in about 1 hour 10 minutes | Servings 20)

Per serving : Calories: 127; Fat: 9g; Carbs: 10.7g; Protein: 2.4g

Ingredients

1 cup cashew butter

1 cup fresh dates, pitted

1/4 cup cocoa powder

1/4 teaspoon ground cloves

1 teaspoon matcha powder

1 teaspoon vanilla extract

1/2 cup hazelnuts, coarsely chopped

Directions

Process all ingredients in your blender until uniform and smooth.

Scrape the batter into a parchment-lined baking sheet. Place it in your freezer for at least 1 hour to set.

Cut into squares and serve. Bon appétit!

Oatmeal Squares with Cranberries

(Ready in about 25 minutes | Servings 20)

Per serving : Calories: 101; Fat: 2.5g; Carbs: 17.2g; Protein: 2.8g

Ingredients

1 ½ cups rolled oats

1/2 cup brown sugar

1 teaspoon baking soda

A pinch of coarse salt

A pinch of grated nutmeg

1/2 teaspoon cinnamon

2/3 cup peanut butter

1 medium banana, mashed

1/3 cup oat milk

1 teaspoon vanilla extract

1/2 cup dried cranberries

Directions

Begin by preheating your oven to 350 degrees F.

In a mixing bowl, thoroughly combine the dry ingredients. In another bowl, combine the wet ingredients.

Then, stir the wet mixture into the dry ingredients; mix to combine well.

Spread the batter mixture in a parchment-lined baking pan. Bake in the preheated oven for about 20 minutes.

Let it cool on a wire rack. Cut into squares and enjoy!

Classic Bread Pudding with Sultanas

(Ready in about 2 hours | Servings 4)

Per serving : Calories: 377; Fat: 6.5g; Carbs: 72g; Protein: 10.7g

Ingredients

10 ounces day-old bread, cut into cubes

2 cups coconut milk

1/2 cup coconut sugar

1 teaspoon vanilla extract

1/2 teaspoon ground cloves

1/2 teaspoon ground cinnamon

1/2 cup Sultanas

Directions

Place the bread cubes in a lightly oiled baking dish.

Now, blend the milk, sugar, vanilla, ground cloves and cinnamon until creamy and smooth.

Spoon the mixture all over the bread cubes, pressing them with a wide spatula to soak well; fold in Sultanas and set aside for about 1 hour.

Bake in the preheated oven at 350 degrees F for about 1 hour or until the top of your pudding is golden brown.

Bon appétit!

Decadent Hazelnut Halvah

(Ready in about 10 minutes | Servings 16)

Per serving : Calories: 169; Fat: 15.5g; Carbs: 6.6g; Protein: 1.9g

Ingredients

1/2 cup tahini

1/2 cup almond butter

1/4 cup coconut oil, melted

4 tablespoons agave nectar

1/2 teaspoon pure almond extract

1/2 teaspoon pure vanilla extract

1/8 teaspoon salt

1/8 teaspoon freshly grated nutmeg

1/2 cup hazelnuts, chopped

Directions

Line a square baking pan with parchment paper.

Mix the ingredients, except for the hazelnuts, until everything is well incorporated.

Scrape the batter into the parchment-lined pan. Press the hazelnuts into the batter.

Place in your freezer until ready to serve. Bon appétit!

Orange Mini Cheesecakes

(Ready in about 10 minutes + chilling time | Servings 12)

Per serving : Calories: 226; Fat: 15.9g; Carbs: 19.8g; Protein: 5.1g

Ingredients

Crust:

1 cup raw almonds

1 cup fresh dates, pitted

Topping:

1/2 cup raw sunflower seeds, soaked overnight and drained

1 cup raw cashew nuts, soaked overnight and drained

1 orange, freshly squeezed

1/4 cup coconut oil, softened

1/2 cup dates, pitted

Garnish:

2 tablespoons caramel topping

Directions

In your food processor, blend the crust ingredients until the mixture comes together; press the crust into a lightly greased muffin tin.

Then, blend the topping ingredients until creamy and smooth. Spoon the topping mixture onto the crust, creating a flat surface with a spatula.

Place these mini cheesecakes in your freezer for about 3 hours. Garnish with caramel topping. Bon appétit!

Berry Compote with Red Wine

(Ready in about 15 minutes | Servings 4)

Per serving : Calories: 260; Fat: 0.5g; Carbs: 64.1g; Protein: 1.1g

Ingredients

4 cups mixed berries, fresh or frozen

1 cup sweet red wine

1 cup agave syrup

1/2 teaspoon star anise

1 cinnamon stick

3-4 cloves

A pinch of grated nutmeg

A pinch of sea salt

Directions

Add all ingredients to a saucepan. Cover with water by 1 inch. Bring to a boil and immediately reduce the heat to a simmer.

Let it simmer for 9 to 11 minutes. Allow it to cool completely.

Bon appétit!

Turkish Irmik Helvasi

(Ready in about 35 minutes | Servings 8)

Per serving : Calories: 349; Fat: 29.1g; Carbs: 18.1g; Protein: 4.7g

Ingredients

1 cup semolina flour

1/2 cup coconut, shredded

1/2 teaspoon baking powder

A pinch of salt

1 teaspoon pure vanilla extract

1 cup vegan butter

1 cup coconut milk

1/2 cup walnuts, ground

Directions

Thoroughly combine the flour, coconut, baking powder, salt and vanilla. Add in the butter and milk; mix to combine.

Fold in the walnuts and let it rest for about 1 hour.

Bake in the preheated oven at 350 degrees F for approximately 30 minutes or until a tester inserted in the center of the cake comes out dry and clean.

Transfer to a wire rack to cool completely before slicing and serving. Bon appétit!

Traditional Greek Koufeto

(Ready in about 15 minutes | Servings 8)

Per serving : Calories: 203; Fat: 6.8g; Carbs: 34.1g; Protein: 3.4g

Ingredients

1 pound pumpkin

8 ounces brown sugar

1 vanilla bean

3-4 cloves

1 cinnamon stick

1 cup almonds, slivered and lightly toasted

Directions

Bring the pumpkin and brown sugar to a boil; add in the vanilla, cloves and cinnamon.

Stir continuously to prevent from sticking.

Cook until your Koufeto has thickened; fold in the almonds; let it cool completely. Enjoy!

Tangy Fruit Salad with Lemon Dressing

(Ready in about 15 minutes | Servings 4)

Per serving : Calories: 223; Fat: 0.8g; Carbs: 56.1g; Protein: 2.4g

Ingredients

Salad:

1/2 pound mixed berries

1/2 pound apples, cored and diced

8 ounces red grapes

2 kiwis, peeled and diced

2 large oranges, peeled and sliced

2 bananas, sliced

Lemon Dressing:

2 tablespoons fresh lemon juice

1 teaspoon fresh ginger, peeled and minced

4 tablespoons agave syrup

Directions

Mix all the ingredients for the salad until well combined.

Then, in a small mixing bowl, whisk all the lemon dressing ingredients.

Dress your salad and serve well chilled. Bon appétit!

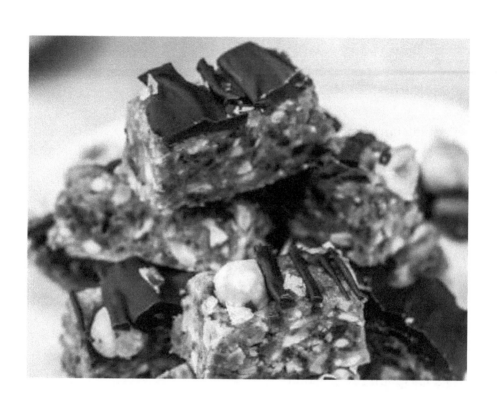

German-Style Apple Crumble

(Ready in about 50 minutes | Servings 8)

Per serving : Calories: 376; Fat: 23.8g; Carbs: 41.3g; Protein: 3.3g

Ingredients

4 apples, cored, peeled and sliced

1/2 cup brown sugar

1 cup all-purpose flour

1/2 cup coconut flour

2 tablespoons flaxseed meal

1 teaspoon baking powder

1/2 teaspoon baking soda

A pinch of sea salt

A pinch of freshly grated nutmeg

1/2 teaspoon ground cinnamon

1/2 teaspoon ground anise

1/2 teaspoon pure vanilla extract

1/2 teaspoon pure coconut extract

1 cup coconut milk

1/2 cup coconut oil, softened

Directions

Arrange the apples on the bottom of a lightly oiled baking pan. Sprinkle brown sugar over them.

In a mixing bowl, thoroughly combine the flour, flaxseed meal, baking powder, baking soda, salt, nutmeg, cinnamon, anise, vanilla and coconut extract.

Add in the coconut milk and softened oil and mix until everything is well incorporated. Spread the topping mixture over the fruit layer.

Bake the apple crumble at 350 degrees F for about 45 minutes or until golden brown. Bon appétit!

Vanilla Cinnamon Pudding

(Ready in about 25 minutes | Servings 4)

Per serving : Calories: 332; Fat: 4.4g; Carbs: 64g; Protein: 9.9g

Ingredients

1 cup basmati rice, rinsed

1 cup water

3 cups almond milk

12 dates, pitted

1 teaspoon vanilla paste

1 teaspoon ground cinnamon

Directions

Add the rice, water and 1 ½ cups of milk to a saucepan. Cover the saucepan and bring the mixture to a boil.

Turn the heat to low; let it simmer for another 10 minutes until all the liquid is absorbed.

Then, add in the remaining ingredients and stir to combine. Let it simmer for 10 minutes more or until the pudding has thickened. Bon appétit!

Mint Chocolate Cake

(Ready in about 45 minutes | Servings 16)

Per serving : Calories: 167; Fat: 7.1g; Carbs: 25.1g; Protein: 1.4g

Ingredients

1/2 cup vegan butter

1/2 cup brown sugar

2 chia eggs

3/4 cup all-purpose flour

1 teaspoon baking powder

A pinch of salt

A pinch of ground cloves

1 teaspoon ground cinnamon

1 teaspoon pure vanilla extract

1/3 cup coconut flakes

1 cup vegan chocolate chunks

A few drops peppermint essential oil

Directions

In a mixing bowl, beat the vegan butter and sugar until fluffy.

Add in the chia eggs, flour, baking powder, salt, cloves, cinnamon and vanilla. Beat to combine well.

Add in the coconut and mix again.

Scrape the mixture into a lightly greased baking pan; bake at 350 degrees F for 35 to 40 minutes.

Melt the chocolate in your microwave and add in the peppermint essential oil; stir to combine well.

Afterwards, spread the chocolate ganache evenly over the surface of the cake. Bon appétit!

Old-Fashioned Cookies

(Ready in about 45 minutes | Servings 12)

Per serving : Calories: 167; Fat: 8.6g; Carbs: 19.6g; Protein: 2.7g

Ingredients

1 cup all-purpose flour

1 teaspoon baking powder

A pinch of salt

A pinch of grated nutmeg

1/2 teaspoon ground cinnamon

1/4 teaspoon ground cardamom

1/2 cup peanut butter

2 tablespoons coconut oil, room temperature

2 tablespoons almond milk

1/2 cup brown sugar

1 teaspoon vanilla extract

1 cup vegan chocolate chips

Directions

In a mixing bowl, combine the flour, baking powder and spices.

In another bowl, combine the peanut butter, coconut oil, almond milk, sugar and vanilla. Stir the wet mixture into the dry ingredients and stir until well combined.

Fold in the chocolate chips. Place the batter in your refrigerator for about 30 minutes. Shape the batter into small cookies and arrange them on a parchment-lined cookie pan.

Bake in the preheated oven at 350 degrees F for approximately 11 minutes. Transfer them to a wire rack to cool slightly before serving. Bon appétit!

Coconut Cream Pie

(Ready in about 15 minutes + chilling time | Servings 12)

Per serving : Calories: 295; Fat: 21.1g; Carbs: 27.1g; Protein: 3.8g

Ingredients

Crust:

2 cups walnuts

10 fresh dates, pitted

2 tablespoons coconut oil at room temperature

1/4 teaspoon groin cardamom

1/2 teaspoon ground cinnamon

1 teaspoon vanilla extract

Filling:

2 medium over-ripe bananas

2 frozen bananas

1 cup full-fat coconut cream, well-chilled

1/3 cup agave syrup

Garnish:

3 ounces vegan dark chocolate, shaved

Directions

In your food processor, blend the crust ingredients until the mixture comes together; press the crust into a lightly oiled baking pan.

Then, blend the filling layer. Spoon the filling onto the crust, creating a flat surface with a spatula.

Transfer the cake to your freezer for about 3 hours. Store in your freezer.

Garnish with chocolate curls just before serving. Bon appétit!

Easy Chocolate Candy

(Ready in about 35 minutes | Servings 8)

Per serving : Calories: 232; Fat: 15.5g; Carbs: 19.6g; Protein: 3.4g

Ingredients

10 ounces dark chocolate, broken into chunks

6 tablespoons coconut milk, warm

1/4 teaspoon ground cinnamon

1/4 teaspoon ground anise

1/2 teaspoon vanilla extract

1/4 cup cacao powder, unsweetened

Directions

Thoroughly combine the chocolate, warm coconut milk, cinnamon, anise and vanilla until everything is well incorporated.

Use a cookie scoop to portion the mixture into 1-ounce portions. Roll the balls with your hands and refrigerate them for at least 30 minutes.

Dip the chocolate balls in the cacao powder and store them in your refrigerator until ready to serve. Bon appétit!

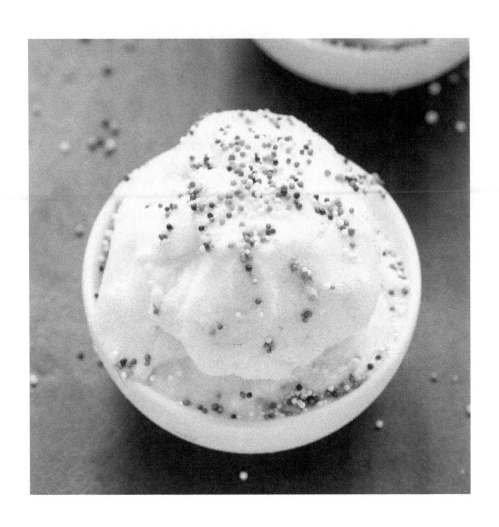

Mom's Raspberry Cobbler

(Ready in about 50 minutes | Servings 7)

Per serving : Calories: 227; Fat: 10.6g; Carbs: 32.1g; Protein: 3.6g

Ingredients

 1 pound fresh raspberries

 1/2 teaspoon fresh ginger, peeled and minced

 1/2 teaspoon lime zest

 2 tablespoons brown sugar

 1 cup all-purpose flour

 1 teaspoon baking powder

 1/4 teaspoon sea salt

 2 ounces agave syrup

 1/4 teaspoon ground cloves

 1/2 teaspoon ground cinnamon

 1/8 teaspoon freshly grated nutmeg

1/2 cup coconut cream

1/2 cup coconut milk

Directions

Arrange the raspberries on the bottom of a lightly oiled baking pan. Sprinkle ginger, lime zest and brown sugar over them.

In a mixing bowl, thoroughly combine the flour, baking powder, salt, agave syrup, ground cloves, cinnamon and nutmeg.

Add in the coconut cream and milk and mix until everything is well incorporated. Spread the topping mixture over the raspberry layer.

Bake your cobbler at 350 degrees F for about 45 minutes or until golden brown. Bon appétit!

Autumn Pear Crisp

(Ready in about 50 minutes | Servings 8)

Per serving : Calories: 289; Fat: 15.4g; Carbs: 35.5g; Protein: 4.4g

Ingredients

4 pears, peeled, cored and sliced

1 tablespoon fresh lemon juice

1/2 teaspoon ground cinnamon

1/2 teaspoon ground anise

1 cup brown sugar

1 ¼ cups quick-cooking oats

1/2 cup water

1/2 teaspoon baking powder

1/2 cup coconut oil, melted

1 teaspoon pure vanilla extract

Directions

Start by preheating your oven to 350 degrees F.

Arrange the pears on the bottom of a lightly oiled baking pan. Sprinkle lemon juice, cinnamon, anise and 1/2 cup of brown sugar over them.

In a mixing bowl, thoroughly combine the quick-cooking oats, water, 1/2 of the brown sugar, baking powder, coconut oil and vanilla extract.

Spread the topping mixture over the fruit layer.

Bake in the preheated oven for about 45 minutes or until golden brown. Bon appétit!

Famous Haystack Cookies

(Ready in about 20 minutes | Servings 9)

Per serving : Calories: 332; Fat: 18.4g; Carbs: 38.5g; Protein: 5.1g

Ingredients

1 cup instant oats

1/2 cup almond butter

2 ounces almonds, ground

1/4 cup cocoa powder, unsweetened

1/2 teaspoon vanilla

1/2 teaspoon ground cinnamon

1/2 teaspoon ground anise

1/4 cup almond milk

3 tablespoons vegan butter

1 cup brown sugar

Directions

In mixing bowl, thoroughly combine the oats, almond butter, ground almonds, cocoa, vanilla, cinnamon and anise; reserve.

In a medium saucepan, bring the milk, butter and sugar to a boil. Let it boil for approximately 1 minute, stirring frequently.

Pour the milk/butter mixture over the oat mixture; stir to combine well.

Drop by teaspoonfuls onto a parchment-lined cookie sheet and let them cool completely. Enjoy!

Double Chocolate Brownies

(Ready in about 25 minutes | Servings 9)

Per serving : Calories: 237; Fat: 14.4g; Carbs: 26.5g; Protein: 2.8g

Ingredients

1/2 cup vegan butter, melted

2 tablespoons applesauce

1/2 cup all-purpose flour

1/2 cup almond flour

1 teaspoon baking powder

2/3 cup brown sugar

1/2 teaspoon vanilla extract

1/3 cup cocoa powder

A pinch of sea salt

A pinch of freshly grated nutmeg

1/4 cup chocolate chips

Directions

Start by preheating your oven to 350 degrees F.

In a mixing bowl, whisk the butter and applesauce until well combined. Then, stir in the remaining ingredients, whisking continuously to combine well.

Pour the batter into a lightly oiled baking pan. Bake in the preheated oven for about 25 minutes or until a tester inserted in the middle comes out clean.

Bon appétit!

Crispy Oat and Pecan Treats

(Ready in about 25 minutes | Servings 10)

Per serving : Calories: 375; Fat: 16.3g; Carbs: 56g; Protein: 4.7g

Ingredients

1 cup all-purpose flour

2 ½ cups instant oats

1 teaspoon baking soda

A pinch of coarse salt

1 cup brown sugar

1/2 cup coconut oil, room temperature

4 tablespoons agave syrup

1 teaspoon vanilla extract

1/4 teaspoon ground cinnamon

1/4 teaspoon ground anise

1/4 teaspoon ground cloves

2 tablespoons applesauce

1/2 cup pecans, roughly chopped

Directions

In a mixing bowl, thoroughly combine the flour, oats, baking soda and salt.

Then, whip the sugar with coconut oil and agave syrup. Add in the spices and applesauce. Add the wet mixture to the dry ingredients.

Fold in the pecans and stir to combine. Spread the batter onto a parchment-lined baking sheet.

Bake your cake at 350 degrees F for about 25 minutes or until the center is set. Let it cool and cut into bars. Bon appétit!

Mom's Raspberry Cheesecake

(Ready in about 15 minutes + chilling time | Servings 9)

Per serving : Calories: 355; Fat: 29.1g; Carbs: 20.1g; Protein: 6.6g

Ingredients

Crust:

1 cup almond flour

1/2 cup macadamia nuts

1 cup dried desiccated coconut

1/2 teaspoon cinnamon

1/4 teaspoon grated nutmeg

Topping:

1 cup raw cashew nuts, soaked overnight and drained

1 cup raw sunflower seeds, soaked overnight and drained

1/4 cup coconut oil, at room temperature

1/2 cup pure agave syrup

1/2 cup freeze-dried raspberries

Directions

In your food processor, blend the crust ingredients until the mixture comes together; press the crust into a lightly greased springform pan.

Then, blend the topping ingredients until creamy and smooth. Spoon the topping mixture onto the crust.

Place the cheesecake in your freezer for about 3 hours. Garnish with some extra raspberries and coconut flakes. Bon appétit!

Chocolate-Glazed Cookies

(Ready in about 45 minutes | Servings 14)

Per serving : Calories: 177; Fat: 12.6g; Carbs: 16.2g; Protein: 1.7g

Ingredients

1/2 cup all-purpose flour

1/2 cup almond flour

1 teaspoon baking powder

A pinch of sea salt

A pinch of grated nutmeg

1/4 teaspoon ground cloves

1/2 cup cocoa powder

1/2 cup cashew butter

2 tablespoons almond milk

1 cup brown sugar

1 teaspoon vanilla paste

4 ounces vegan chocolate

1 ounce coconut oil

Directions

In a mixing bowl, combine the flour, baking powder, salt, nutmeg, cloves and cocoa powder.

In another bowl, combine the cashew butter, almond milk, sugar and vanilla paste. Stir the wet mixture into the dry ingredients and stir until well combined.

Place the batter in your refrigerator for about 30 minutes. Shape the batter into small cookies and arrange them on a parchment-lined cookie pan.

Bake in the preheated oven at 330 degrees F for approximately 10 minutes. Transfer the pan to a wire rack to cool slightly.

Microwave the chocolate until melted; mix the melted chocolate with the coconut oil. Spread the glaze over your cookies and let it cool completely. Bon appétit!

Caramel Bread Pudding

(Ready in about 2 hours | Servings 5)

Per serving : Calories: 386; Fat: 7.3g; Carbs: 69.3g; Protein: 10.8g

Ingredients

12 ounces stale bread, cut into cubes

3 cups almond milk

1/2 cup agave syrup

1/4 teaspoon coarse salt

1/4 teaspoon freshly grated nutmeg

1 teaspoon pure vanilla extract

1/2 teaspoon ground cinnamon

1 cup almonds, slivered

1 cup caramel sauce

Directions

Place the bread cubes in a lightly oiled baking dish.

Now, blend the milk, agave syrup, coarse salt, freshly grated nutmeg, vanilla extract and cinnamon until creamy and smooth.

Spoon the mixture all over the bread cubes, pressing them with a wide spatula to soak well; fold in the almonds and set aside for about 1 hour.

Bake in the preheated oven at 350 degrees F for about 1 hour or until the top of your pudding is golden brown.

Spoon the caramel sauce over the bread pudding and serve at room temperature. Bon appétit!

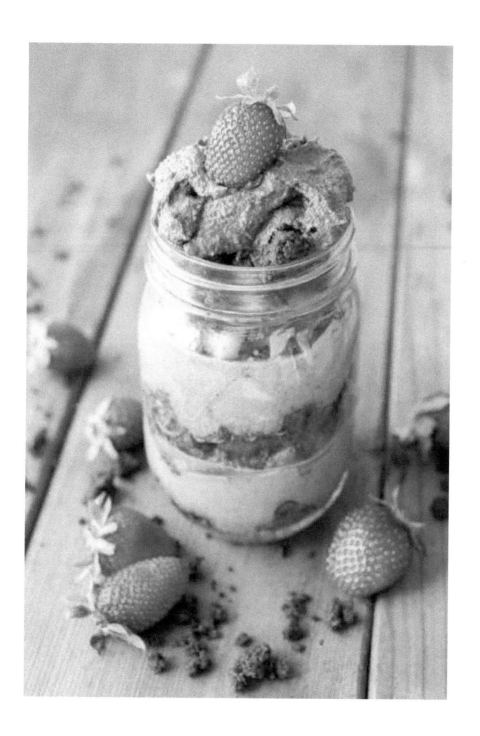

The Best Granola Bars Ever

(Ready in about 25 minutes | Servings 16)

Per serving : Calories: 227; Fat: 12.8g; Carbs: 25.5g; Protein: 3.7g

Ingredients

1 cup vegan butter

1 cup rolled oats

1 cup all-purpose flour

1 cup oat flour

1 teaspoon baking powder

A pinch of coarse sea salt

A pinch of freshly grated nutmeg

1/4 teaspoon ground cloves

1/4 teaspoon ground cardamom

1/4 teaspoon ground cinnamon

1 heaping cup packed dates, pitted

4 ounces raspberry preserves

Directions

Begin by preheating your oven to 350 degrees F.

In a mixing bowl, thoroughly combine the dry ingredients. In another bowl, combine the wet ingredients.

Then, stir the wet mixture into the dry ingredients; mix to combine well.

Spread the batter mixture in a parchment-lined baking pan. Bake in the preheated oven for about 20 minutes.

Let it cool on a wire rack and then, cut into bars. Bon appétit!

Old-Fashioned Fudge Penuche

(Ready in about 15 minutes | Servings 12)

Per serving : Calories: 156; Fat: 11.1g; Carbs: 13.6g; Protein: 1.5g

Ingredients

4 ounces dark vegan chocolate

1/2 cup almond milk

1 cup brown sugar

1/4 cup coconut oil, softened

1/2 cup walnuts, chopped

1/4 teaspoon ground cloves

1/2 teaspoon ground cinnamon

Directions

Microwave the chocolate until melted.

In a saucepan, heat the milk and add the warm milk to the melted chocolate.

Add in the remaining ingredients and mix to combine well.

Pour the mixture into a well-greased pan and place it in your refrigerator until set. Bon appétit

(Ready in about 10 minutes + chilling time | Servings 12)

Per serving : Calories: 235; Fat: 17.8g; Carbs: 17.5g; Protein: 4.6g

Ingredients

1 cup almonds, ground

1 ½ cups dates, pitted

1 ½ cups vegan cream cheese

1/4 cup coconut oil, softened

1/2 cup fresh or frozen blueberries

Directions

In your food processor, blend the almonds and 1 cup of dates until the mixture comes together; press the crust into a lightly greased muffin tin.

Then, blend the remaining 1/2 cup of dates along with the vegan cheese, coconut oil and blueberries until creamy and smooth. Spoon the topping mixture onto the crust.

Place these mini cheesecakes in your freezer for about 3 hours. Bon appétit!

Spiced Cauliflower Bites

(Ready in about 25 minutes | Servings 4)

Per serving : Calories: 187; Fat: 4.1g; Carbs: 32.8g; Protein: 6.2g

Ingredients

1 pound cauliflower florets

1 cup all-purpose flour

1 tablespoon olive oil

1 tablespoon tomato paste

1 teaspoon onion powder

1 teaspoon garlic powder

1 teaspoon smoked paprika

1/2 teaspoon dried oregano

1/2 teaspoon dried basil

1/4 cup hot sauce

Directions

Begin by preheating your oven to 450 degrees F. Pat the cauliflower florets dry using a kitchen towel.

Mix the remaining ingredients until well combined. Dip the cauliflower florets in the batter until well coated on all sides.

Place the cauliflower florets in a parchment-lined baking pan.

Roast for about 25 minutes or until cooked through. Bon appétit!

Swiss-Style Potato Cake (Rösti)

(Ready in about 25 minutes | Servings 5)

Per serving : Calories: 204; Fat: 11g; Carbs: 24.6g; Protein: 2.9g

Ingredients

1 ½ pounds russets potatoes, peeled, grated and squeezed

1 teaspoon coarse sea salt

1/2 teaspoon red pepper flakes, crushed

1/2 teaspoon freshly ground black pepper

4 tablespoons olive oil

Directions

Mix the grated potatoes, salt, red pepper and ground black pepper.

Heat the oil in a cast-iron skillet.

Drop handfuls of the potato mixture into the skillet.

Cook your potato cake over medium for about 10 minutes. Cover the potatoes and cook for another 10 minutes until the bottom of the potato cake is golden brown. Bon appétit!

Creamed Vegan "Tuna" Salad

(Ready in about 10 minutes | Servings 8)

Per serving : Calories: 252; Fat: 18.4g; Carbs: 17.1g; Protein: 5.5g

Ingredients

2 (15-ounce) cans chickpeas, rinsed

3/4 cup vegan mayonnaise

1 teaspoon brown mustard

1 small red onion, chopped

2 pickles, chopped

1 teaspoon capers, drained

1 tablespoon fresh parsley, chopped

1 tablespoon fresh coriander, chopped

Sea salt and ground black pepper, to taste

2 tablespoons sunflower seeds, roasted

Directions

Mix all the ingredients until everything is well incorporated.

Place your salad in the refrigerator until ready to serve.

Bon appétit!

Traditional Hanukkah Latkes

(Ready in about 30 minutes | Servings 6)

Per serving : Calories: 283; Fat: 18.4g; Carbs: 27.3g; Protein: 3.2g

Ingredients

1 ½ pounds potatoes, peeled, grated and drained

3 tablespoons green onions, sliced

1/3 cup all-purpose flour

1/2 teaspoon baking powder

1/2 teaspoon sea salt, preferably kala namak

1/4 teaspoon ground black pepper

1/2 olive oil

5 tablespoons applesauce

1 tablespoon fresh dill, roughly chopped

Directions

Thoroughly combine the grated potato, green onion, flour, baking powder, salt and black pepper.

Preheat the olive oil in a frying pan over a moderate heat.

Spoon 1/4 cup of potato mixture into the pan and cook your latkes until golden brown on both sides. Repeat with the remaining batter.

Serve with applesauce and fresh dill. Bon appétit!

Thanksgiving Herb Gravy

(Ready in about 20 minutes | Servings 6)

Per serving : Calories: 165; Fat: 1.6g; Carbs: 33.8g; Protein: 6.8g

Ingredients

3 cups vegetable broth

1 ½ cups brown rice, cooked

6 ounces Cremini mushrooms, chopped

1 teaspoon dried basil

1 teaspoon dried oregano

1/2 teaspoon dried rosemary

1/2 teaspoon dried thyme

1/2 teaspoon garlic, minced

1/4 cup unsweetened plain almond milk

Sea salt and freshly ground black pepper

Directions

Bring the vegetable broth to a boil over medium-high heat; add in the rice and mushrooms and reduce the heat to a simmer.

Let it simmer for about 12 minutes, until the mushrooms have softened. Remove from the heat.

Then, blend the mixture until creamy and uniform.

Add the remaining ingredients and heat your gravy over medium heat until everything is cooked through.

Serve with mashed potatoes or vegetables of choice. Bon appétit!

Grandma's Cornichon Relish

(Ready in about 15 minutes + chilling time | Servings 9)

Per serving : Calories: 45; Fat: 0g; Carbs: 10.2g; Protein: 0.3g

Ingredients

3 cups cornichon, finely chopped

1 cup white onion, finely chopped

1 teaspoon sea salt

1/3 cup distilled white vinegar

1/4 teaspoon mustard seeds

1/3 cup sugar

1 tablespoon arrowroot powder, dissolved in 1 tablespoon water

Directions

Place the cornichon, onion and salt in a sieve set over a bowl; drain for a few hours. Squeeze out as much liquid as possible.

Bring the vinegar, mustard seeds and sugar to a boil; add in the 1/3 teaspoon of the sea salt and let it boil until the sugar has dissolved.

Add in the cornichon-onion mixture and continue to simmer for 2 to 3 minutes more. Stir in the arrowroot powder mixture and continue to simmer for 1 to 2 minutes more.

Transfer the relish to a bowl and place, uncovered, in your refrigerator for about 2 hours. Bon appétit!

Apple and Cranberry Chutney

(Ready in about 1 hour | Servings 7)

Per serving : Calories: 208; Fat: 0.3g; Carbs: 53g; Protein: 0.6g

Ingredients

1 ½ pounds cooking apples, peeled, cored and diced

1/2 cup sweet onion, chopped

1/2 cup apple cider vinegar

1 large orange, freshly squeezed

1 cup brown sugar

1 teaspoon fennel seeds

1 tablespoon fresh ginger, peeled and grated

1 teaspoon sea salt

1/2 cup dried cranberries

Directions

In a saucepan, place the apples, sweet onion, vinegar, orange juice, brown sugar, fennel seeds, ginger and salt. Bring the mixture to a boil.

Immediately turn the heat to simmer; continue to simmer, stirring occasionally, for approximately 55 minutes, until most of the liquid has absorbed.

Set aside to cool and add in the dried cranberries. Store in your refrigerator for up to 2 weeks.

Bon appétit!

Homemade Apple Butter

(Ready in about 35 minutes | Servings 16)

Per serving : Calories: 106; Fat: 0.3g; Carbs: 27.3g; Protein: 0.4g

Ingredients

5 pounds apples, peeled, cored and diced

1 cup water

2/3 cup granulated brown sugar

1 tablespoon ground cinnamon

1 teaspoon ground cloves

1 tablespoon vanilla essence

A pinch of freshly grated nutmeg

A pinch of salt

Directions

Add the apples and water to a heavy-bottomed pot and cook for about 20 minutes.

Then, mash the cooked apples with a potato masher; stir the sugar, cinnamon, cloves, vanilla, nutmeg and salt into the mashed apples; stir to combine well.

Continue to simmer until the butter has thickened to your desired consistency.

Bon appétit!

Homemade Peanut Butter

(Ready in about 5 minutes | Servings 16)

Per serving : Calories: 144; Fat: 9.1g; Carbs: 10.6g; Protein: 6.9g

Ingredients

1 ½ cups peanuts, blanched

A pinch of coarse salt

1 tablespoons agave syrup

Directions

In your food processor or a high-speed blender, pulse the peanuts until ground. Then, process for 2 minutes more, scraping down the sides and bottom of the bowl.

Add in the salt and agave syrup.

Run your machine for another 2 minutes or until your butter is completely creamy and smooth.

Bon appétit!

Roasted Pepper Spread

(Ready in about 10 minutes | Servings 10)

Per serving : Calories: 111; Fat: 6.8g; Carbs: 10.8g; Protein: 4.4g

Ingredients

2 red bell peppers, roasted and seeded

1 jalapeno pepper, roasted and seeded

4 ounces sun-dried tomatoes in oil, drained

2/3 cup sunflower seeds

2 tablespoons onion, chopped

1 garlic clove

1 tablespoon Mediterranean herb mix

Sea salt and ground black pepper, to taste

1/2 teaspoon turmeric powder

1 teaspoon ground cumin

2 tablespoons tahini

Directions

Place all the ingredients in the bowl of your blender or food processor.

Process until creamy, uniform and smooth.

Store in an airtight container in your refrigerator for up to 2 weeks. Bon appétit!

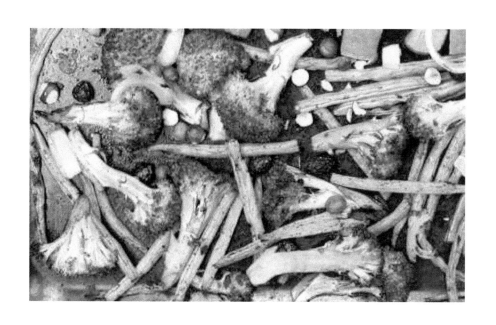

Classic Vegan Butter

(Ready in about 10 minutes | Servings 16)

Per serving : Calories: 89; Fat: 10.1g; Carbs: 0.2g; Protein: 0.1g

Ingredients

2/3 cup refined coconut oil, melted

1 tablespoon sunflower oil

1/4 cup soy milk

1/2 teaspoon malt vinegar

1/3 teaspoon coarse sea salt

Directions

Add the coconut oil, sunflower oil, milk and vinegar to the bowl of your blender. Blitz to combine well.

Add in the sea salt and continue to blend until creamy and smooth; refrigerate until set.

Bon appétit!

Mediterranean-Style Zucchini Pancakes

(Ready in about 20 minutes | Servings 4)

Per serving : Calories: 260; Fat: 14.1g; Carbs: 27.1g; Protein: 4.6g

Ingredients

1 cup all-purpose flour

1/2 teaspoon baking powder

1/2 teaspoon dried oregano

1/2 teaspoon dried basil

1/2 teaspoon dried rosemary

Sea salt and ground black pepper, to taste

1 ½ cups zucchini, grated

1 chia egg

1/2 cup rice milk

1 teaspoon garlic, minced

2 tablespoons scallions, sliced

4 tablespoons olive oil

Directions

Thoroughly combine the flour, baking powder and spices. In a separate bowl, combine the zucchini, chia egg, milk, garlic and scallions.

Add the zucchini mixture to the dry flour mixture; stir to combine well.

Then, heat the olive oil in a frying pan over a moderate flame. Cook your pancakes for 2 to 3 minutes per side until golden brown.

Bon appétit!

Traditional Norwegian Flatbread (Lefse)

(Ready in about 20 minutes | Servings 7)

Per serving : Calories: 215; Fat: 4.5g; Carbs: 38.3g; Protein: 5.6g

Ingredients

3 medium-sized potatoes

1/2 cup all-purpose flour

1/2 cup besan

Sea salt, to taste

1/4 teaspoon ground black pepper

1/2 teaspoon cayenne pepper

2 tablespoons olive oil

Directions

Boil the potatoes in a lightly salted water until they've softened.

Peel and mash the potatoes and then, add in the flour, besan and spices.

Divide the dough into 7 equal balls. Roll out each ball on a little floured work surface.

Heat the olive oil in a frying pan over medium-low heat and cook each flatbread for 2 to 3 minutes. Serve immediately.

Bon appétit!

Basic Cashew Butter

(Ready in about 20 minutes | Servings 12)

Per serving : Calories: 130; Fat: 10.1g; Carbs: 6.8g; Protein: 3.8g

Ingredients

3 cups raw cashew nuts

1 tablespoon coconut oil

Directions

In your food processor or a high-speed blender, pulse the cashew nuts until ground. Then, process them for 5 minutes more, scraping down the sides and bottom of the bowl.

Add in the coconut oil.

Run your machine for another 10 minutes or until your butter is completely creamy and smooth. Enjoy!

Apple and Almond Butter Balls

(Ready in about 15 minutes | Servings 12)

Per serving : Calories: 134; Fat: 2.4g; Carbs: 27.6g; Protein: 2.3g

Ingredients

1/2 cup almond butter

1 cup apple butter

1/3 cup almonds

1 cup fresh dates, pitted

1/2 teaspoon ground cinnamon

1/4 teaspoon ground cardamom

1/2 teaspoon almond extract

1/2 teaspoon rum extract

2 ½ cups old-fashioned oats

Directions

Place the almond butter, apple butter, almonds, dates and spices in the bowl of your blender or food processor.

Process the mixture until you get a thick paste.

Stir in the oats and pulse a few more times to blend well. Roll the mixture into balls and serve well-chilled.

Raw Mixed Berry Jam

(Ready in about 1 hour 5 minutes | Servings 10)

Per serving : Calories: 57; Fat: 1.6g; Carbs: 10.7g; Protein: 1.3g

Ingredients

1/4 pound fresh raspberries

1/4 pound fresh strawberries, hulled

1/4 pound fresh blackberries

2 tablespoons lemon juice, freshly squeezed

10 dates, pitted

3 tablespoons chia seeds

Directions

Puree all the ingredients in your blender or food processor.

Let it sit for about 1 hour, stirring periodically.

Store your jam in sterilized jars in your refrigerator for up to 4 days. Bon appétit!

Basic Homemade Tahini

(Ready in about 10 minutes | Servings 16)

Per serving : Calories: 135; Fat: 13.4g; Carbs: 2.2g; Protein: 3.6g

Ingredients

10 ounces sesame seeds, hulled

3 tablespoons canola oil

1/4 teaspoon kosher salt

Directions

Toast the sesame seeds in a nonstick skillet for about 4 minutes, stirring continuously. Cool the sesame seeds completely.

Transfer the sesame seeds to the bowl of your food processor. Process for about 1 minute.

Add in the oil and salt and process for a further 4 minutes, scraping down the bottom and sides of the bowl.

Store your tahini in the refrigerator for up to 1 month. Bon appétit!

Homemade Vegetable Stock

(Ready in about 55 minutes | Servings 6)

Per serving : Calories: 68; Fat: 4.4g; Carbs: 6.2g; Protein: 0.8g

Ingredients

2 tablespoons olive oil

1 cup onion, chopped

2 cup carrots, chopped

1 cup celery, chopped

4 cloves garlic, minced

2 sprigs rosemary, chopped

2 sprigs thyme, chopped

1 bay laurel

1 teaspoon mixed peppercorns

Sea salt, to taste

6 cups water

Directions

In a heavy-bottomed pot, heat the oil over medium-high heat. Now, sauté the vegetables for about 10 minutes, stirring periodically to ensure even cooking.

Add in the garlic and spices and continue sautéing for 1 minute or until aromatic.

Add in the water, turn the heat to a simmer and let it cook for a further 40 minutes.

Set a strainer over a big bowl and line it with cheesecloth. Pour the stock through and discard the solids.

Bon appétit!

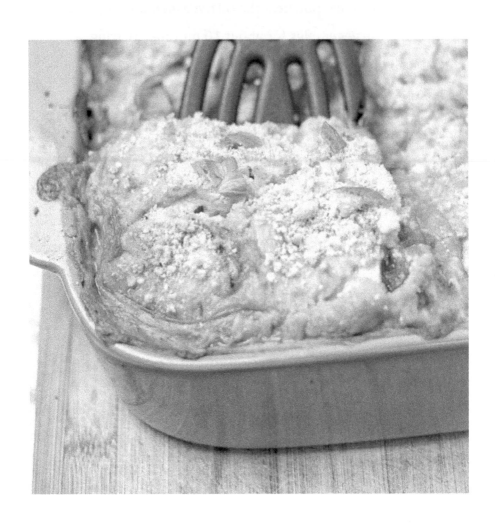

10-Minute Basic Caramel

(Ready in about 10 minutes | Servings 10)

Per serving : Calories: 183; Fat: 7.7g; Carbs: 30g; Protein: 0g

Ingredients

1/4 cup coconut oil

1 ½ cups granulated sugar

1/3 teaspoon coarse sea salt

1/3 cup water

2 tablespoons almond butter

Directions

Melt the coconut oil and sugar in a saucepan for 1 minute.

Whisk in the remaining ingredients and continue to cook until everything is fully incorporated and your caramel is deeply golden.

Bon appétit!

Nutty Chocolate Fudge Spread

(Ready in about 25 minutes | Servings 16)

Per serving : Calories: 207; Fat: 20.4g; Carbs: 5.4g; Protein: 4.6g

Ingredients

1 pound walnuts

1 ounce coconut oil, melted

2 tablespoons corn flour

4 tablespoons cocoa powder

A pinch of grated nutmeg

1/3 teaspoon ground cinnamon

A pinch of salt

Directions

Roast the walnuts in the preheated oven at 350 degrees F for approximately 10 minutes until your walnuts are fragrant and lightly browned.

In your food processor or a high-speed blender, pulse the walnuts until ground. Then, process them for 5 minutes more, scraping down the sides and bottom of the bowl; reserve.

Melt the coconut oil over medium heat. Add in the corn flour and continue to cook until the mixture starts to boil.

Turn the heat to a simmer, add in the cocoa powder, nutmeg, cinnamon and salt; continue to cook, stirring occasionally, for about 10 minutes.

Fold in the ground walnuts, stir to combine and store in a glass jar. Enjoy!

Cashew Cream Cheese

(Ready in about 10 minutes | Servings 6)

Per serving : Calories: 197; Fat: 14.4g; Carbs: 11.4g; Protein: 7.4g

Ingredients

1 ½ cups cashews, soaked overnight and drained

1/3 cup water

1/4 teaspoon coarse sea salt

1/4 teaspoon dried dill weed

1/4 teaspoon garlic powder

2 tablespoons nutritional yeast

2 probiotic capsules

Directions

Process the cashews and water in your blender until creamy and uniform.

Add in the salt, dill, garlic powder and nutritional yeast; continue to blend until everything is well incorporated.

Spoon the mixture into a sterilized glass jar. Add in the probiotic powder and combine with a wooden spoon (not metal!)

Cover the jar with a clean kitchen towel and let it stand on the kitchen counter to ferment for 24-48 hours.

Keep in your refrigerator for up to a week. Bon appétit!

Homemade Chocolate Milk

(Ready in about 10 minutes | Servings 4)

Per serving : Calories: 79; Fat: 3.1g; Carbs: 13.3g; Protein: 1.3g

Ingredients

4 teaspoons cashew butter

4 cups water

1/2 teaspoon vanilla paste

4 teaspoons cocoa powder

8 dates, pitted

Directions

Place all the ingredients in the bowl of your high-speed blender.

Process until creamy, uniform and smooth.

Keep in a glass bottle in your refrigerator for up to 4 days. Enjoy!

Traditional Korean Buchimgae

(Ready in about 20 minutes | Servings 4)

Per serving : Calories: 315; Fat: 19g; Carbs: 26.1g; Protein: 9.5g

Ingredients

1/2 cup all-purpose flour

1/2 cup chickpea flour

1/2 teaspoon baking powder

1 teaspoon garlic powder

1/4 teaspoon ground cumin

1/2 teaspoon sea salt

1 carrot, trimmed and grated

1 small onion, finely chopped

1 cup Kimchi

1 green chili, minced

1 flax egg

1 tablespoon bean paste

1 cup rice milk

4 tablespoons canola oil

Directions

Thoroughly combine the flour, baking powder and spices. In a separate bowl, combine the carrot, onion, Kimchi, green chili, flax egg, bean paste and rice milk.

Add the vegetable mixture to the dry flour mixture; stir to combine well.

Then, heat the oil in a frying pan over a moderate flame. Cook the Korean pancakes for 2 to 3 minutes per side until crispy.

Bon appétit!

Easy Homemade Nutella

(Ready in about 25 minutes | Servings 20)

Per serving : Calories: 187; Fat: 17.1g; Carbs: 7g; Protein: 4g

Ingredients

3 ½ cups hazelnuts

1 teaspoon vanilla seeds

A pinch of coarse sea salt

A pinch of grated nutmeg

1/2 teaspoon ground cinnamon

1/2 teaspoon ground cardamom

1 cup dark chocolate chips

Directions

Roast the hazelnuts in the preheated oven at 350 degrees F for approximately 13 minutes until your hazelnuts are fragrant and lightly browned.

In your food processor or a high-speed blender, pulse the hazelnuts until ground. Then, process the mixture for 5 minutes more, scraping down the sides and bottom of the bowl.

Add in the remaining ingredients.

Run your machine for a further 4 to 5 minutes or until the mixture is completely creamy and smooth. Enjoy!

Delicious Lemon Butter

(Ready in about 10 minutes | Servings 8)

Per serving : Calories: 87; Fat: 3.4g; Carbs: 14.6g; Protein: 0g

Ingredients

1/2 cup granulated sugar

2 tablespoons cornstarch

1/2 teaspoon lemon zest, grated

1 cup water

2 tablespoons fresh lemon juice

2 tablespoons coconut oil

Directions

In a saucepan, combine the sugar, cornstarch and lemon zest over a moderate heat.

Stir in the water and lemon juice and continue to cook until the mixture has thickened. Heat off.

Stir in the coconut oil. Bon appétit!

Mom's Blueberry Jam

(Ready in about 40 minutes | Servings 20)

Per serving : Calories: 108; Fat: 0.1g; Carbs: 27.6g; Protein: 0.2g

Ingredients

1 ½ pounds fresh blueberries

1 pound granulated sugar

1 cinnamon stick

5-6 cloves

1 vanilla pod, split lengthways

1 lemon, juiced

Directions

Mix all the ingredients in a saucepan.

Continue to cook over medium heat, stirring constantly, until the sauce has reduced and thickened for about 30 minutes.

Remove from the heat. Leave your jam to sit for 10 minutes. Ladle into sterilized jars and cover with the lids. Let it cool completely.

Bon appétit!

Authentic Spanish Tortilla

(Ready in about 30 minutes | Servings 4)

Per serving : Calories: 365; Fat: 13.9g; Carbs: 48.1g; Protein: 14.5g

Ingredients

2 tablespoons olive oil

1 ½ pounds russet potatoes, peeled and sliced

1 onion, chopped

Sea salt and ground black pepper, to taste

1/4 cup rice milk

8 ounces tofu, pressed and drained

1/2 cup besan

2 tablespoons cornstarch

1/2 teaspoon ground cumin

1/4 teaspoon ground allspice

Directions

Heat 1 tablespoon of the olive oil in a frying pan. Then, add the potatoes, onion, salt and black pepper to the frying pan.

Cook for about 20 minutes or until the potatoes have softened.

In a mixing bowl, thoroughly combine the remaining ingredients. Add in the potato mixture and stir to combine.

Heat the remaining 1 tablespoon of the olive oil in a frying pan over medium-low heat. Cook your tortilla for 5 minutes per side. Serve warm.

Bon appétit!

Traditional Belarusian Draniki

(Ready in about 30 minutes | Servings 4)

Per serving : Calories: 350; Fat: 14.4g; Carbs: 45.6g; Protein: 6.8g

Ingredients

4 waxy potatoes, peeled, grated and squeezed

4 tablespoons scallions, chopped

1 green chili pepper, chopped

1 red chili pepper, chopped

1/3 cup besan

1/2 teaspoon baking powder

1 teaspoon paprika

Sea salt and red pepper, to taste

1/4 cup canola oil

2 tablespoons fresh cilantro, chopped

Directions

Thoroughly combine the grated potatoes, scallions, pepper, besan, baking powder, paprika, salt and red pepper.

Preheat the oil in a frying pan over a moderate heat.

Spoon 1/4 cup of potato mixture into the pan and cook your draniki until golden brown on both sides. Repeat with the remaining batter.

Serve with fresh cilantro. Bon appétit!

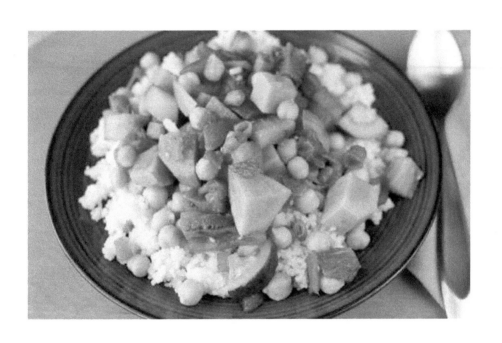

Mediterranean Tomato Gravy

(Ready in about 20 minutes | Servings 6)

Per serving : Calories: 106; Fat: 6.6g; Carbs: 9.6g; Protein: 0.8g

Ingredients

3 tablespoons olive oil

1 red onion, chopped

3 cloves garlic, crushed

4 tablespoons cornstarch

1 can (14 ½-ounce) tomatoes, crushed

1/2 teaspoon dried basil

1/2 teaspoon dried oregano

1/2 teaspoon dried thyme

1 teaspoon dried parsley flakes

Sea salt and black pepper, to taste

Directions

Heat the olive oil in a large saucepan over medium-high heat. Once hot, sauté the onion and garlic until tender and fragrant.

Add in the cornstarch and continue to cook for 1 minute more.

Add in the canned tomatoes and bring to a boil over medium-high heat; stir in the spices and turn the heat to a simmer.

Let it simmer for about 10 minutes until everything is cooked through.

Serve with vegetables of choice. Bon appétit!

Pepper and Cucumber Relish

(Ready in about 20 minutes + chilling time | Servings 10)

Per serving : Calories: 66; Fat: 0.3g; Carbs: 15.3g; Protein: 1.5g

Ingredients

6 cucumbers, chopped

1 red bell pepper, seeded and chopped

1 green bell pepper, seeded and chopped

2 tablespoons coarse sea salt

1/2 cup wine vinegar

2/3 cup granulated sugar

1/2 teaspoon fennel seeds

1/4 teaspoon mustard seeds

1/4 teaspoon ground turmeric

1/2 teaspoon ground allspice

1 tablespoon mixed peppercorns

4 teaspoons cornstarch

Directions

Place the cucumber, bell pepper and salt in a sieve set over a bowl; drain for a few hours. Squeeze out as much liquid as possible.

Bring the vinegar and sugar to a boil; add in the 1/3 teaspoon of the sea salt and let it boil until the sugar has dissolved.

Add in the cucumber-pepper mixture and continue to simmer for 2 to 3 minutes more. Stir in the spices and cornstarch; continue to simmer for 1 to 2 minutes more.

Transfer the relish to a bowl and place, uncovered, in your refrigerator for about 2 hours. Bon appétit!

Homemade Almond Butter

(Ready in about 20 minutes | Servings 20)

Per serving : Calories: 131; Fat: 11.3g; Carbs: 4.8g; Protein: 4.8g

Ingredients

1 pound almonds

A pinch of sea salt

A pinch of grated nutmeg

Directions

Roast the almonds in the preheated oven at 350 degrees F for approximately 9 minutes until your nuts are fragrant and lightly browned.

In your food processor or a high-speed blender, pulse the almonds until ground. Then, process the mixture for 5 minutes more, scraping down the sides and bottom of the bowl.

Add in the salt and nutmeg.

Run your machine for another 10 minutes or until your butter is completely creamy and smooth. Enjoy!

Indian-Style Mango Chutney

(Ready in about 1 hour | Servings 7)

Per serving : Calories: 273; Fat: 2.3g; Carbs: 64.3g; Protein: 2.4g

Ingredients

5 mangoes, peeled and diced

1 yellow onion, chopped

2 red chilies, chopped

3/4 cup balsamic vinegar

1 ½ cups granulated sugar

1 teaspoon coriander seeds

1 tablespoon chana dal

1/2 teaspoon jeera

1/4 teaspoon turmeric powder

1/4 teaspoon Himalayan salt

1/2 cup currants

Directions

In a saucepan, place the mangoes, onion, red chilies, vinegar, granulated sugar, coriander seeds, chana dal, jeera, turmeric powder and salt. Bring the mixture to a boil.

Immediately turn the heat to simmer; continue to simmer, stirring occasionally, for approximately 55 minutes, until most of the liquid has absorbed.

Set aside to cool and add in the currants. Store in your refrigerator for up to 2 weeks.

Bon appétit!

Easy Vegetable Pajeon

(Ready in about 20 minutes | Servings 4)

Per serving : Calories: 255; Fat: 10.6g; Carbs: 33.3g; Protein: 6.2g

Ingredients

1/2 cup all-purpose flour

1/2 cup potato starch

1 teaspoon baking powder

1/3 teaspoon Himalayan salt

1/2 cup kimchi, finely chopped

4 scallions, chopped

1 carrot, trimmed and chopped

2 bell peppers, chopped

1 green chili pepper, chopped

1 cup kimchi liquid

2 tablespoons olive oil

Dipping sauce:

2 tablespoons soy sauce

2 teaspoons rice vinegar

1 teaspoon fresh ginger, finely grated

Directions

Thoroughly combine the flour, potato starch, baking powder and salt. In a separate bowl, combine the vegetables and kimchi liquid.

Add the vegetable mixture to the dry flour mixture; stir to combine well.

Then, heat the oil in a frying pan over a moderate flame. Cook the Pajeon for 2 to 3 minutes per side until crispy.

Meanwhile, mix the sauce ingredients. Serve your Pajeon with the sauce for dipping. Bon appétit!

Healthy Chocolate Peanut Butter

(Ready in about 15 minutes | Servings 20)

Per serving : Calories: 118; Fat: 9.2g; Carbs: 6.9g; Protein: 5.1g

Ingredients

2 ½ cups peanuts

1/2 teaspoon coarse sea salt

1/2 teaspoon cinnamon powder

1/2 cup cocoa powder

10 dates, pitted

Directions

Roast the peanuts in the preheated oven at 350 degrees F for approximately 7 minutes until the peanuts are fragrant and lightly browned.

In your food processor or a high-speed blender, pulse the peanuts until ground. Then, process the mixture for 2 minutes more, scraping down the sides and bottom of the bowl.

Add in the salt, cinnamon, cocoa powder and dates.

Run your machine for another 2 minutes or until your butter is completely creamy and smooth. Enjoy!

Chocolate Walnut Spread

(Ready in about 20 minutes | Servings 15)

Per serving : Calories: 78; Fat: 4.7g; Carbs: 9g; Protein: 1.5g

Ingredients

1 cup walnuts

1 teaspoon pure vanilla extract

1/2 cup agave nectar

4 tablespoons cocoa powder

A pinch of ground cinnamon

A pinch of grated nutmeg

A pinch of sea salt

4 tablespoons almond milk

Directions

Roast the walnuts in the preheated oven at 350 degrees F for approximately 10 minutes until they are fragrant and lightly browned.

In your food processor or a high-speed blender, pulse the walnuts until ground. Then, process the mixture for 5 minutes more, scraping down the sides and bottom of the bowl.

Add in the remaining ingredients.

Run your machine for a further 5 minutes or until the mixture is completely creamy and smooth. Enjoy!

Pecan and Apricot Butter

(Ready in about 15 minutes | Servings 16)

Per serving : Calories: 163; Fat: 17g; Carbs: 2.5g; Protein: 1.4g

Ingredients

2 ½ cups pecans

1/2 cup dried apricots, chopped

1/2 cup sunflower oil

1 teaspoon bourbon vanilla

1/4 teaspoon ground anise

1/2 teaspoon cinnamon

1/8 teaspoon grated nutmeg

1/8 teaspoon salt

Directions

In your food processor or a high-speed blender, pulse the pecans until ground. Then, process the pecans for 5 minutes more, scraping down the sides and bottom of the bowl.

Add in the remaining ingredients.

Run your machine for a further 5 minutes or until the mixture is completely creamy and smooth. Enjoy!

Cinnamon Plum Preserves

(Ready in about 40 minutes | Servings 20)

Per serving : Calories: 223; Fat: 0.3g; Carbs: 58.1g; Protein: 0.8g

Ingredients

5 pounds ripe plums rinsed

2 pounds granulated sugar

2 tablespoons lemon juice

3 cinnamon sticks

Directions

Mix all the ingredients in a saucepan.

Continue to cook over medium heat, stirring constantly, until the sauce has reduced and thickened for about 30 minutes.

Remove from the heat. Leave your jam to sit for 10 minutes. Ladle into sterilized jars and cover with the lids. Let it cool completely.

Bon appétit!

Middle-Eastern Tahini Spread

(Ready in about 10 minutes | Servings 16)

Per serving : Calories: 143; Fat: 13.3g; Carbs: 6.2g; Protein: 3.9g

Ingredients

10 ounces sesame seeds

3 tablespoons cocoa powder

1 teaspoon vanilla seeds

1/4 teaspoon kosher salt

1/2 cup fresh dates, pitted

3 tablespoons coconut oil

Directions

Toast the sesame seeds in a nonstick skillet for about 4 minutes, stirring continuously. Cool the sesame seeds completely.

Transfer the sesame seeds to the bowl of your food processor. Process for about 1 minute.

Add in the remaining ingredients and process for a further 4 minutes, scraping down the bottom and sides of the bowl.

Store your tahini spread in the refrigerator for up to 1 month. Bon appétit!

Vegan Ricotta Cheese

(Ready in about 10 minutes | Servings 12)

Per serving : Calories: 74; Fat: 6.3g; Carbs: 3.3g; Protein: 2.7g

Ingredients

1/2 cup raw cashew nuts, soaked overnight and drained

1/2 cup raw sunflower seeds, soaked overnight and drained

1/4 cup water

1 heaping tablespoon coconut oil, melted

1 tablespoon lime juice, freshly squeezed

1 tablespoon white vinegar

1/4 teaspoon Dijon mustard

2 tablespoons nutritional yeast

1/2 teaspoon garlic powder

1/2 teaspoon turmeric powder

1/2 teaspoon salt

Directions

Process the cashews, sunflower seeds and water in your blender until creamy and uniform.

Add in the remaining ingredients; continue to blend until everything is well incorporated.

Keep in your refrigerator for up to a week. Bon appétit!

Super Easy Almond Milk

(Ready in about 10 minutes | Servings 6)

Per serving : Calories: 78; Fat: 6g; Carbs: 4.8g; Protein: 2.5g

Ingredients

1 cup raw almonds, soaked overnight and drained

6 cups water

1 tablespoon maple syrup

A pinch of grated nutmeg

A pinch of salt

A pinch of ground cinnamon

1 teaspoon vanilla extract

Directions

Place all the ingredients in the bowl of your high-speed blender.

Process until creamy, uniform and smooth.

Strain the liquid using a nut milk bag; squeeze until all of the liquid is extracted.

Keep in a glass bottle in your refrigerator for up to 4 days. Enjoy!

Homemade Vegan Yogurt

(Ready in about 10 minutes | Servings 6)

Per serving : Calories: 141; Fat: 14.2g; Carbs: 4g; Protein: 1.3g

Ingredients

1 ½ cups full-fat coconut milk

1 teaspoon maple syrup

A pinch of coarse sea salt

2 capsules vegan probiotic

Directions

Spoon the coconut milk into a sterilized glass jar. Add in the maple syrup and salt.

Empty your probiotic capsules and stir with a wooden spoon (not metal!)

Cover the jar with a clean kitchen towel and let it stand on the kitchen counter to ferment for 24-48 hours.

Keep in your refrigerator for up to a week. Bon appétit!

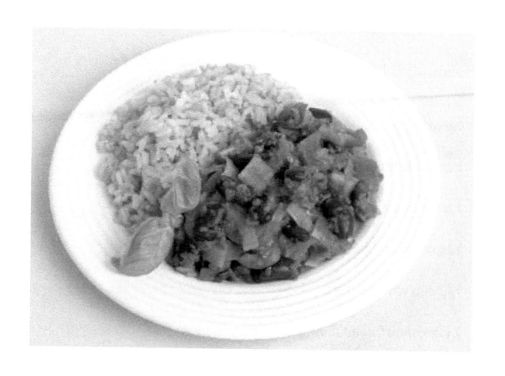

South Asian Masala Paratha

(Ready in about 20 minutes | Servings 5)

Per serving : Calories: 441; Fat: 30.4g; Carbs: 38.1g; Protein: 5.2g

Ingredients

2 cups all-purpose flour

1 teaspoon Kala namak salt

1/2 teaspoon garam masala

1/2 cup warm water

1 tablespoon canola oil

10 tablespoons coconut oil, softened

Directions

In a mixing bowl, thoroughly combine the flour, salt and garam masala. Make a well in the flour mixture and gradually add in the water and canola oil; mix to combine.

Knead the dough until it forms a sticky ball. Let it rest in your refrigerator overnight.

Divide the dough into 5 equal balls and roll them out on a clean surface. Spread the coconut oil all over the paratha and fold it in half. Spread the coconut oil over it and fold it again.

Roll each paratha into a circle approximately 8 inches in diameter.

Heat a griddle until hot. Cook each paratha for about 3 minutes or until bubbles form on the surface. Turn over and cook on the other side for 3 minutes longer. Serve warm.

Traditional Swedish Raggmunk

(Ready in about 30 minutes | Servings 5)

Per serving : Calories: 356; Fat: 22.1g; Carbs: 36.5g; Protein: 4.3g

Ingredients

1 ½ pounds waxy potatoes, peeled, grated and squeezed

3 tablespoons shallots, chopped

2 chia eggs

1/2 cup all-purpose flour

1 teaspoon baking powder

Sea salt and ground black, to season

1 teaspoon cayenne pepper

1/2 cup canola oil

6 tablespoons applesauce

Directions

Thoroughly combine the grated potatoes, shallots, chia eggs, flour, baking powder, salt, black pepper and cayenne pepper.

Preheat the oil in a frying pan over a moderate heat.

Spoon 1/4 cup of the potato mixture into the pan and cook the potato cakes for about 5 minutes per side. Repeat with the remaining batter.

Serve with applesauce and enjoy!

Buffalo Gravy with Beer

(Ready in about 30 minutes | Servings 5)

Per serving : Calories: 222; Fat: 16.8g; Carbs: 11.2g; Protein: 7.3g

Ingredients

3 tablespoons olive oil

1 small red onion, chopped

1 teaspoon garlic, minced

1/3 cup whole wheat flour

3 cups vegetable broth

1/2 teaspoon dried rosemary

1/2 teaspoon dried oregano

1/2 teaspoon dried parsley flakes

1/2 teaspoon dried sage

1 teaspoon hot paprika

Sea salt and freshly cracked black peppercorns, to taste

1 cup beer

Directions

Heat the olive oil in a large saucepan over medium-high heat. Once hot, sauté the onion and garlic until tender and fragrant.

Add in the flour and continue to cook for 1 minute more.

Pour in the vegetable broth and bring to a boil over medium-high heat; stir in the spices and turn the heat to a simmer.

Pour in the beer and let it simmer, partially covered, for about 10 minutes until everything is cooked through.

Serve with mashed potatoes or cauliflower. Bon appétit!

Spicy Cilantro and Mint Chutney

(Ready in about 10 minutes | Servings 9)

Per serving : Calories: 15; Fat: 0g; Carbs: 0.9g; Protein: 0.1g

Ingredients

1 ½ bunches fresh cilantro

6 tablespoons scallions, sliced

3 tablespoons fresh mint leaves

2 jalapeno peppers, seeded

1/2 teaspoon kosher salt

2 tablespoons fresh lime juice

1/3 cup water

Directions

Place all the ingredients in the bowl of your blender or food processor.

Then, combine the ingredients until your desired consistency has been reached.

Bon appétit!

Cinnamon Almond Butter

Ready in about 30 minutes | Servings 16)

Per serving : Calories: 118; Fat: 8.9g; Carbs: 7.5g; Protein: 3.8g

Ingredients

2 cups almonds

1 tablespoon cinnamon, ground

1 teaspoon pure vanilla extract

3 tablespoons agave syrup

A pinch of sea salt

A pinch of grated nutmeg

Directions

Roast the almonds in the preheated oven at 350 degrees F for approximately 9 minutes until your nuts are fragrant and lightly browned.

In your food processor or a high-speed blender, pulse the almonds until ground. Then, process the mixture for 10 minutes more, scraping down the sides and bottom of the bowl.

Add in the cinnamon, vanilla, agave syrup, salt and nutmeg.

Run your machine for another 10 minutes or until your butter is completely creamy and smooth. Enjoy!

Rainbow Vegetable Pancakes

(Ready in about 20 minutes | Servings 4)

Per serving : Calories: 222; Fat: 4.9g; Carbs: 38.1g; Protein: 7.5g

Ingredients

1 cup all-purpose flour

1 teaspoon baking powder

Sea salt and ground black pepper, to taste

1 teaspoon paprika

1 cup zucchini, grated

1 cup button mushrooms, chopped

2 medium carrots, trimmed and grated

1 red onion, finely chopped

1 garlic clove, minced

1 cup spinach, torn into pieces

1/4 cup water

1 teaspoon hot sauce

2 chia eggs

Directions

Thoroughly combine the flour, baking powder, salt, black pepper and paprika. In a separate bowl, combine the vegetables and water.

Add in the hot sauce and chia eggs and mix to combine well. Add the vegetable mixture to the dry flour mixture; stir to combine well.

Then, heat the oil in a frying pan over a moderate flame. Cook the pancakes for 2 to 3 minutes per side until crispy and golden brown.

Bon appétit!

Garden Tomato Relish

(Ready in about 10 minutes + chilling time | Servings 10)

Per serving : Calories: 208; Fat: 21.8g; Carbs: 3.5g; Protein: 0.7g

Ingredients

1 pound tomatoes, chopped

1 red onion, chopped

1 garlic clove, minced

1 cup extra-virgin olive oil

2 tablespoons capers

1 teaspoon chili powder

1 tablespoon curry powder

2 tablespoons cilantro, chopped

2 tablespoons malt vinegar

Directions

Thoroughly combine the tomatoes, onion, garlic and olive oil. Grill for about 8 minutes.

Add in the remaining ingredients and stir to combine well.

Transfer the relish to a bowl and place, uncovered, in your refrigerator for about 2 hours. Bon appétit!

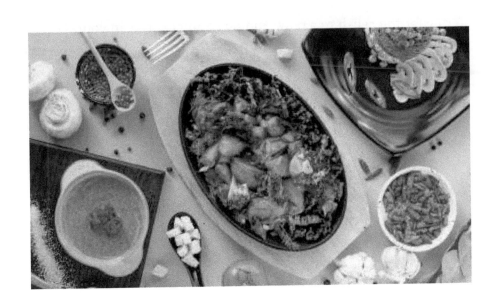

Crunchy Peanut Butter

(Ready in about 10 minutes | Servings 20)

Per serving : Calories: 114; Fat: 9g; Carbs: 5.6g; Protein: 4.8g

Ingredients

2 ½ cups peanuts

1/2 teaspoon coarse sea salt

1/2 teaspoon cinnamon powder

10 dates, pitted

Directions

Roast the peanuts in the preheated oven at 350 degrees F for approximately 7 minutes until the peanuts are fragrant and lightly browned.

In your food processor or a high-speed blender, pulse the peanuts until ground. Reserve for about 1/2 cup of the mixture.

Then, process the mixture for 2 minutes more, scraping down the sides and bottom of the bowl.

Add in the salt, cinnamon and dates.

Run your machine for another 2 minutes or until your butter is smooth. Add in the reserved peanuts and stir with a spoon. Enjoy!

Easy Orange Butter

(Ready in about 10 minutes | Servings 7)

Per serving : Calories: 140; Fat: 13.6g; Carbs: 6.3g; Protein: 0g

Ingredients

2 tablespoons granulated sugar

2 tablespoons cornstarch

1 teaspoon orange zest

1 teaspoon fresh ginger, peeled and minced

2 tablespoons orange juice

1/2 cup water

A pinch of grated nutmeg

A pinch of grated kosher salt

7 tablespoons coconut oil, softened

Directions

In a saucepan, combine the sugar, cornstarch, orange zest and ginger over a moderate heat.

Stir in the orange juice, water, nutmeg and salt; continue to cook until the mixture has thickened. Heat off.

Stir in the coconut oil. Bon appétit!